John Oakson

I REMEMBER THE 1950s

Good Old Days History for Seniors

seniorality

Table of Contents

Welcome to the 1950s

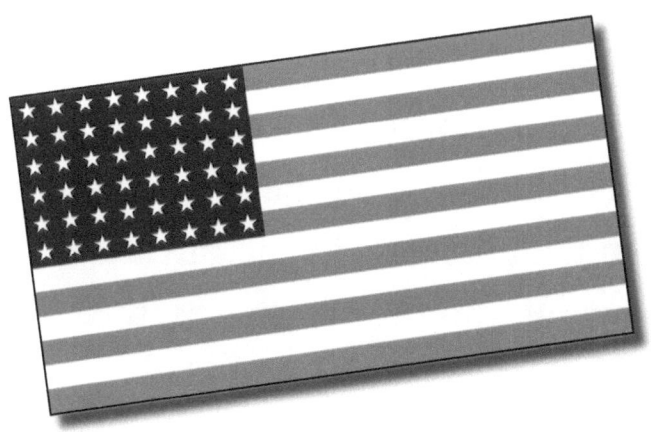

Step into our time machine, and let's take a journey back to the fabulous 1950s! It was a time of poodle skirts, Elvis Presley, and rock and roll, a decade filled with fascinating stories and big changes.

Imagine a country bouncing back from the hardships of World War II. The 1950s in the United States were a time of remarkable economic growth. Factories buzzed with activity, and the construction of new houses seemed endless. Thanks to the GI Bill, more people could get an education and buy homes, leading to an era of suburban living that defined the American dream.

But the '50s wasn't just about economic prosperity. It was also a time of the "baby boom," with a sudden increase in the birthrate. Families were growing, and the nation was, too.

In the background, a cold wind was blowing - the Cold War. The United States and the Soviet Union were locked in a fierce rivalry, and the fear of communism swept the nation. Senator Joseph McCarthy led a campaign of suspicion known as the Red Scare, where people feared communist infiltration into American society and politics.

In the midst of all this, something extraordinary was happening on the civil rights front. In 1954, the Supreme Court declared segregation in public schools unconstitutional with the landmark Brown v. Board of Education decision. A year later, a woman named Rosa Parks refused to give up her bus seat in Montgomery, Alabama, sparking the Montgomery Bus Boycott. The civil rights movement was gaining steam.

Television was becoming a household staple. Iconic shows like "I Love Lucy," "The Ed Sullivan Show," and "The Honeymooners" kept families entertained. And don't forget the birth of rock and roll music with Elvis Presley, whose hip-shaking moves drove the nation wild.

The 1950s marked the beginning of the space race, and it all began with the launch of Sputnik, the first artificial satellite, by the Soviet Union in 1957. The U.S. responded with a newfound interest in space exploration, leading to the Apollo program and that incredible moon landing in 1969.

Women were navigating a shifting landscape. Many returned to traditional roles as homemakers, but beneath the surface, something was brewing. Betty Friedan questioned the "cult of domesticity," and the concept of the "feminine mystique" was taking root, laying the foundation for the women's rights movement of the '60s.

Technological advances were happening left and right. The first credit card was introduced, the microchip was invented, and the interstate highway system was expanding, making it easier for families to hit the road for adventures.

Beyond U.S. borders, the nation was involved in international affairs. The Korean War raged on, and NATO was established to keep the world secure. In Iran, the U.S. played a role in the overthrow of Prime Minister Mohammad Mosaddegh, which had significant geopolitical consequences.

July 4, 1959 saw the Stars and Stripes change from 48 to 49 stars to represent the new state of Alaska.

The 1950s was a time of change, progress, and challenges. It set the stage for the cultural and social transformations of the '60s, but it's also remembered for the incredible music, exciting technological breakthroughs, and the birth of the American dream in the suburbs. The '50s had its ups and downs, but it was certainly a decade to remember!

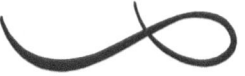

America's Dynamic Leaders - Presidents

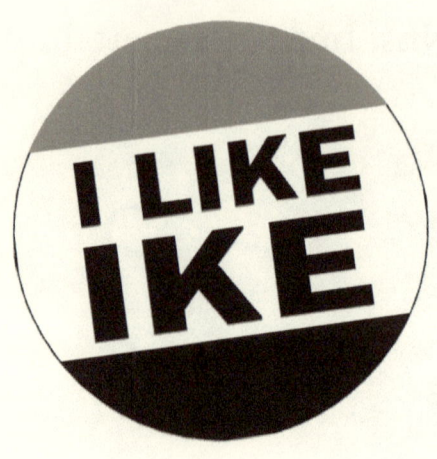

The 1950s were an incredibly transformative period in American history. With World War II behind them, the United States was charting a new course, and at the helm were a trio of remarkable Presidents who navigated the nation through post-war challenges, the early days of the Cold War, and a rapidly changing society.

Let's take a friendly stroll down memory lane and get to know the leaders who guided the nation through this eventful decade.

Harry S. Truman -
The Commander-in-Chief

Our journey begins with Harry S. Truman, a Missourian who became the 33rd President of the United States. Truman, a Democrat, faced the daunting task of transitioning the nation from the devastation of World War II to a time of peace and reconstruction. He was the man behind some pivotal decisions, including the controversial but ultimately game-changing atomic bombings of Hiroshima and Nagasaki.

Truman's leadership also gave birth to the United Nations and the Marshall Plan, a massive economic aid package that helped war-ravaged Europe get back on its feet. His down-to-earth demeanor and famous "The buck stops here" sign on his desk resonated with the American people, who saw him as a trustworthy and resolute leader.

Dwight D. Eisenhower - The War Hero Turned President

In 1952, the nation turned to a beloved war hero and the Supreme Commander of the Allied Expeditionary Forces during World War II, General Dwight D. Eisenhower. As a Republican, Eisenhower came into office with an air of optimism, promising a new beginning. His famous campaign slogan, "I Like Ike," captured the hearts of Americans.

Eisenhower's tenure, often referred to as the "Eisenhower Era," was marked by domestic tranquility and economic growth. He balanced the nation's desire for peace with the need for military preparedness in the face of the Cold War. His Eisenhower Doctrine pledged U.S. support to Middle Eastern nations threatened by communism, and he took a strong stance on civil rights by enforcing desegregation in the public schools.

Eisenhower's leadership gave America a sense of stability and a respite from the tumultuous years that preceded his presidency.

John F. Kennedy - A New Generation of Hope

As the 1950s turned into the 1960s, the nation was ready for fresh, youthful leadership, and they found it in John F. Kennedy. Kennedy, a charismatic young senator from Massachusetts, was elected as the 35th President in 1960.

His administration ushered in a new era of activism and hope, characterized by ambitious space exploration programs, the promise of civil rights, and the Peace Corps, which encouraged Americans to volunteer and serve abroad.

Kennedy's famous words, "Ask not what your country can do for you; ask what you can do for your country," still resonate today, reflecting the spirit of his time. He aimed to address pressing issues such as the Cuban Missile Crisis, and he inspired Americans with his vision for a better future.

The 1950s presidents, Truman, Eisenhower, and the dawning Kennedy era, played integral roles in guiding the United States through a time of post-war recovery, civil rights challenges, and global conflicts. Their leadership styles and legacies continue to influence the course of our nation's history and stand as a testament to the resilience and adaptability of America during transformative times.

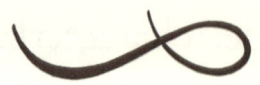

Born into a Brighter Tomorrow - The Baby Boom

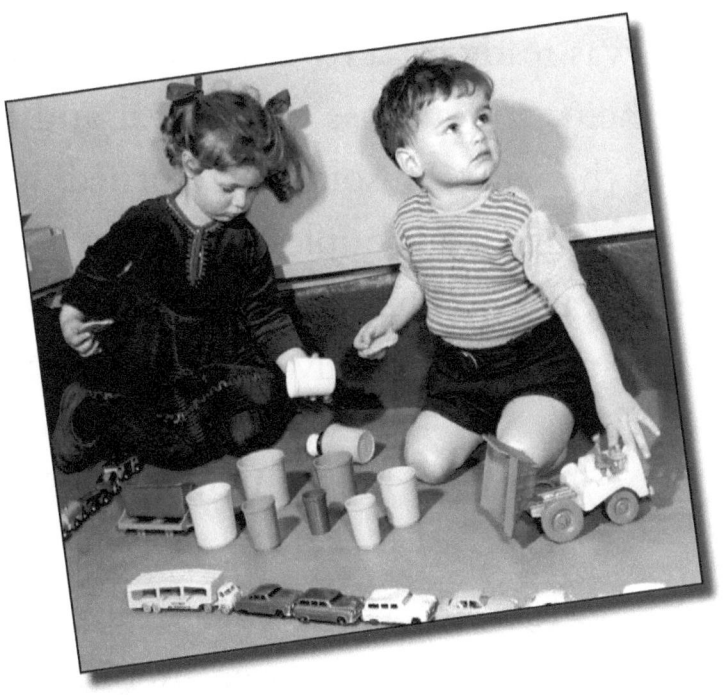

Ah, the Baby Boom. The post-World War II era was filled with optimism, economic prosperity, and the joyful sound of newborns cooing in nurseries. This was the decade when America celebrated life by welcoming a generation that would come to be known as the Baby Boomers.

A Time of Renewal and Hope

After the tumultuous years of World War II, America was ready for a fresh start. The war was behind them, and a sense of renewal and hope hung in the air. As soldiers returned home, families reunited, and couples started envisioning their post-war lives, they had one thing in mind: embracing the joys of family and parenthood.

The Baby Boom Arrives

Between 1946 and 1964, the United States experienced a remarkable surge in births. The highest birth rates were seen in the mid-1950s, and this extraordinary generation of Baby Boomers was born. Families across the nation grew as couples eagerly welcomed their little bundles of joy.

Changing Family Dynamics

The Baby Boom had a profound impact on family dynamics. Households were becoming larger, and the ideal image of the loving family with a mom, dad, and kids became a cherished reality. It was a time when family bonds were strengthened, and the importance of togetherness was embraced with open arms.

Economic Prosperity and Modern Living

The 1950s weren't just about babies; it was a time of unparalleled economic prosperity and the rise of consumerism. Families had more disposable income, and they eagerly embraced the modern conveniences and technological wonders of the era. Televisions, automobiles, and state-of-the-art household appliances became staples in every home.

Opportunity and Education

One of the key factors that contributed to the Baby Boom was the GI Bill. This post-war program offered veterans educational and housing benefits, opening doors to higher education and vocational training. It helped create a more educated and skilled workforce, fostering a sense of optimism and opportunity for young families.

Living the Suburban Dream

Suburban life became a dream come true for many Baby Boomer families. Suburbs blossomed around major cities, offering spacious and peaceful living. Here, children could play in the yard, ride their bikes on quiet streets, and families could enjoy the comfort of a home with a white picket fence.

Cultural Impact

As the Baby Boomers grew and matured, they left an indelible mark on American culture. They embraced the music and spirit of rock and roll, became key players in the civil rights movement, and championed social change in the 1960s and 1970s. Their impact was transformative, and their legacy continues to shape American society.

The Baby Boom Legacy

The Baby Boom was more than just a demographic shift; it was a cultural and social phenomenon. The spirit of optimism and the celebration of life in the 1950s played a pivotal role in defining the Baby Boomer generation. As they continue to influence and lead in the 21st century, their legacy remains a testament to the enduring vitality of a generation that was truly born out of hope and possibility.

So, let's raise a toast to the Baby Boomers and the vibrant, hopeful 1950s era that welcomed them into the world—a generation that shaped history with their dynamism, diversity, and optimism.

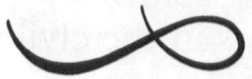

Chilly Waters -
The Cold War and the Red Scare

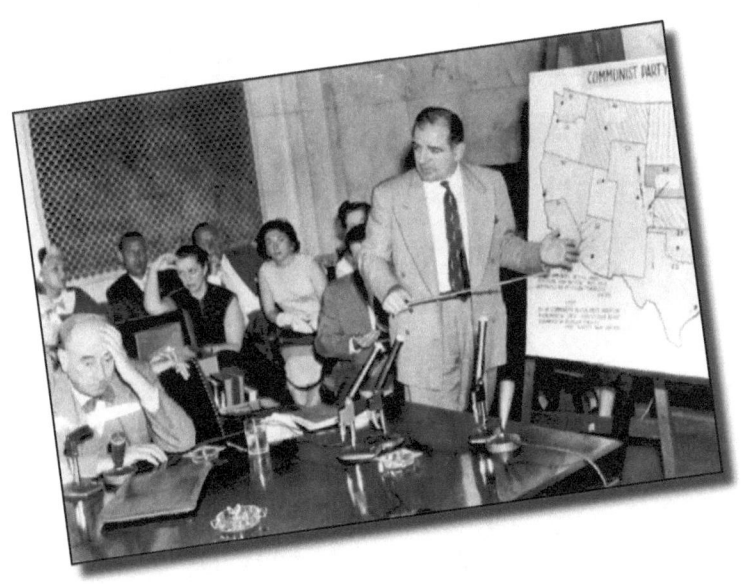

Picture this: the 1950s in the United States—a time of sock hops, drive-in movies, and American optimism. But beneath the surface, there was another narrative playing out, one that would come to define the era—the Cold War and the Red Scare. Let's delve into this chapter of history, marked by tension and suspicion, and explore how Americans found themselves in uncharted territory during this intriguing decade.

The Cold War Chill

The end of World War II ushered in a new global dynamic, the Cold War. It was a time when the United States and the Soviet Union, two superpowers with opposing ideologies, engaged in a geopolitical and ideological struggle for supremacy. The specter of nuclear conflict hung heavily over the world.

The Domino Effect of Communism

During the Cold War, the fear of communism and the spread of Soviet influence was pervasive. The U.S. believed that the fall of one country to communism could lead to a domino effect, with neighboring nations also adopting the ideology. As a result, the U.S. sought to contain communism and prevent its spread.

The Red Scare Takes Hold

One of the most notable features of this era was the Red Scare, characterized by fear and suspicion of communism. Senator Joseph McCarthy emerged as a central figure in the Red Scare. He conducted investigations and hearings, accusing individuals in the government, Hollywood, and various sectors of society of being communist sympathizers or spies. It was a time of deep suspicion and allegations that led to damaged reputations and ruined careers.

McCarthyism and HUAC

The House Un-American Activities Committee (HUAC) played a significant role in the Red Scare, conducting investigations and hearings to root out communism. Artists, writers, and intellectuals were often called before the committee, facing the choice of revealing names of suspected communists or facing blacklisting from their professions.

Hollywood and the Blacklist

The entertainment industry was not immune to the Red Scare's reach. The Hollywood Ten, a group of screenwriters, directors, and producers, refused to cooperate with HUAC, leading to their imprisonment and the introduction of the Hollywood blacklist. Many in the industry found their careers derailed, and some lived in fear of being labeled as communist sympathizers.

The McCarran Internal Security Act

In 1950, Congress passed the McCarran Internal Security Act, which required communist organizations to register with the government. It also allowed for the detention of suspected subversives in case of a national emergency. The act reflected the pervasive fear of communism during this time.

A Period of Tension and Change

The Cold War and the Red Scare had a profound impact on American society. It was a time of tension, suspicion, and conformity. The fear of communism influenced politics, culture, and even individual lives. The era also gave birth to a culture of conformity, as people sought to avoid being labeled as communist sympathizers.

Legacy of the Cold War and the Red Scare

The Cold War eventually thawed, but the legacy of this era still lingers. The fear of communism and the impact of McCarthyism on individuals and the entertainment industry serve as a reminder of the power of fear and the importance of safeguarding civil liberties.

In the end, the 1950s, though a time of great promise and cultural vibrancy, were also marked by the shadow of the Cold War and the Red Scare. It was a period of contrasts and challenges, where the pursuit of American ideals sometimes led down unexpected paths. Yet, through it all, it remains a chapter in American history that continues to provoke reflection and discussion about the balance between security and individual freedoms.

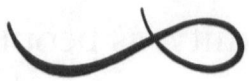

Reaching for the Stars - The Space Race

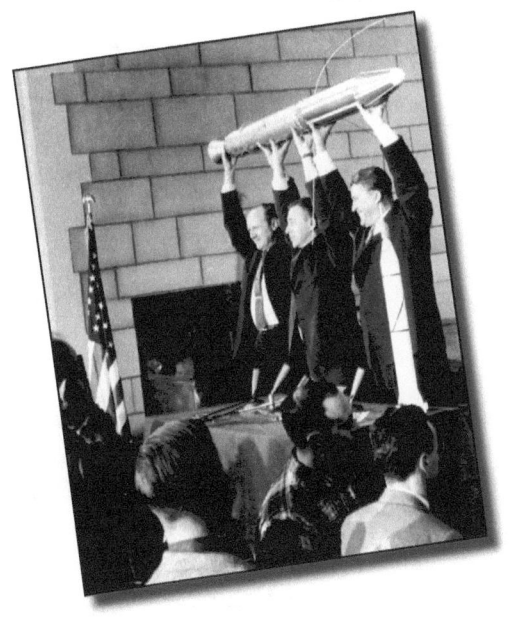

Forget rock 'n' roll, something truly out-of-this-world was taking shape in 1950s America—the Space Race. It was a time when the imagination soared, and the stars above beckoned, as the United States embarked on a thrilling journey to conquer the cosmos. Join us as we relive the excitement of this remarkable era when the race to space was on, and the possibilities seemed endless.

The Roots of the Space Race

The post-World War II era saw the dawn of the Cold War, and with it came the competition between the United States and the Soviet Union for global supremacy. The Space Race was a technological and ideological battle, with both nations striving to demonstrate their scientific prowess.

Sputnik and the Shock of the Century

In 1957, the Soviet Union sent shockwaves around the world when it launched Sputnik, the first artificial satellite. This beeping, metal sphere in the sky sent a clear message: the Soviets had taken the lead in space exploration. The American response was a mix of amazement, anxiety, and determination.

NASA Takes Flight

To catch up and surpass the Soviet Union, the United States established the National Aeronautics and Space Administration (NASA) in 1958. It was the birth of a new era in space exploration. Under NASA's guidance, the Mercury and Gemini programs laid the groundwork for what would become the Apollo program.

The Mercury Seven and Astronaut Heroes

The Mercury program, which ran from 1958 to 1963, was America's first human spaceflight program. It featured the "Mercury Seven," a group of seven brave astronauts who captured the nation's imagination. Names like John Glenn, Alan Shepard, and Gus Grissom became household heroes, and their daring missions became symbols of American courage and exploration.

Technological Advances and the Space Legacy

The Space Race brought about extraordinary technological advancements. New materials, computing technology, and life support systems were developed, many of which had far-reaching applications beyond space exploration.

Inspiration for the Future

The Space Race was more than a mere rivalry; it was a symbol of human potential and the unyielding spirit of exploration. It inspired generations of scientists, engineers, and dreamers. Today, it continues to shape the way we view our place in the universe.

Looking back, we're reminded of a time when the sky was not the limit but merely the beginning. It was an era that embraced the impossible and proved that with determination and innovation, we could reach for the stars. The legacy of the

Space Race lives on, inspiring the dreamers and stargazers of tomorrow to continue pushing the boundaries of human achievement.

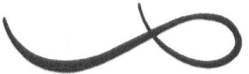

City Lights to Picket Fences – Suburbanization

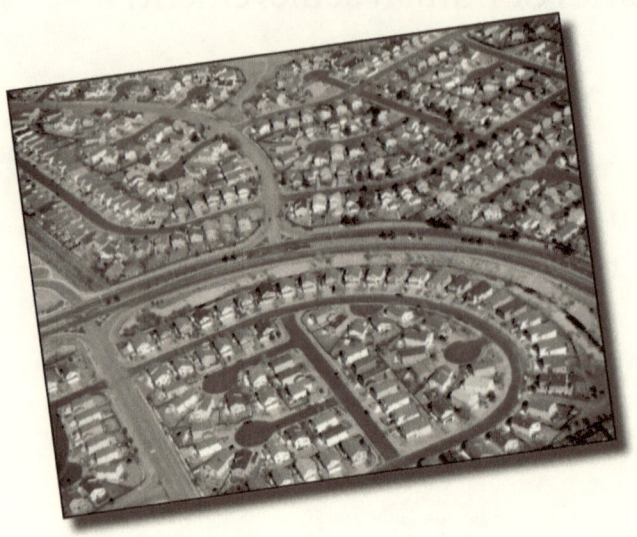

Let's take a leisurely stroll down the tree-lined streets of the 1950s—a time when suburbs were the embodiment of the American dream. It was an era when the bustling city gave way to quiet neighborhoods with white picket fences, and the concept of suburban living became synonymous with the pursuit of a happy and harmonious family life. Join us as we explore the rise of suburbanization in 1950s America, where communities flourished, dreams were built, and the spirit of family reigned supreme.

Post-War Promise

The end of World War II marked the beginning of a new chapter in American history. The country was eager to leave behind the scars of war and embrace the possibilities of peace. The post-war economic boom provided the perfect backdrop for suburbanization.

Levittown and the Birth of Mass-Produced Suburbs

Levittown, New York, is often seen as the birthplace of the modern American suburb. In 1947, William Levitt began constructing rows of nearly identical homes, each with a charming lawn and a white picket fence. These homes were not just houses; they were the promise of a fresh start, affordable living, and a piece of the American dream.

The Baby Boom and Growing Families

As we know, the 1950s were also marked by the Baby Boom, with families across the nation welcoming an abundance of children. Suburbs provided the perfect setting for these growing families, offering more space, yards to play in, and safety away from the city's hustle and bustle.

The Suburban Ideal

Suburban living embodied a specific ideal—a life of tranquility, safety, and community. It was a place where neighbors knew each other, where children rode their bikes on quiet streets, and where the American dream could be pursued with a sense of serenity. The suburbs offered proximity to the city for work while providing a serene retreat for family life.

Car Culture and Commuting

The suburbs and the automobile went hand in hand. The expansion of highways and the affordability of cars made commuting to work in the city a feasible option. This allowed families to enjoy the best of both worlds—a peaceful suburban existence with easy access to urban amenities.

The Rise of Shopping Centers and Malls

Shopping also underwent a transformation in the 1950s. Strip malls and enclosed shopping centers began to dot the suburban landscape. This era saw the rise of the suburban shopping mall, creating new destinations for families to gather and enjoy leisure time.

The Legacy of Suburbanization

The 1950s saw a profound shift in the American way of life. The rise of suburbanization changed the nation's landscape and influenced the trajectory of family life. It was a time when communities flourished, neighborly bonds were formed, and the dream of owning a home with a white picket fence was within reach for many.

Today, the legacy of suburbanization lives on. Suburban communities have evolved, yet the idea of a peaceful and family-friendly life remains central to the American experience. Suburbanization in the 1950s was more than a housing trend; it was the embodiment of an enduring vision—a place where families could thrive, children could play, and dreams could come to life amid the comforting embrace of a suburban landscape.

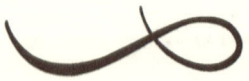

Turning the Tide -
The Civil Rights Movement

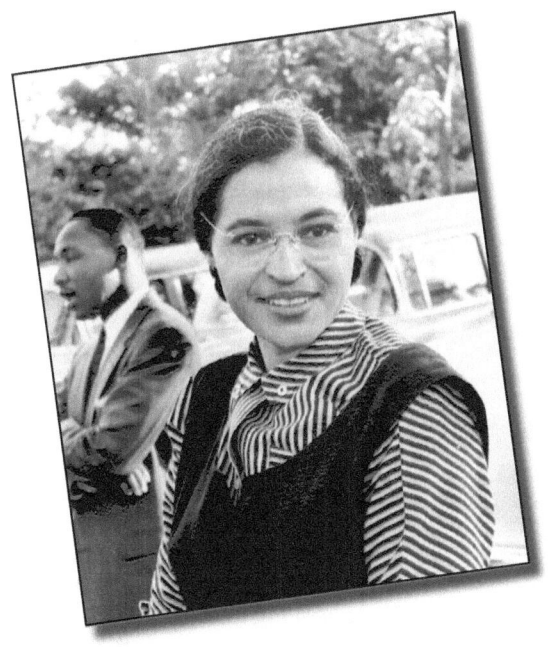

Something important happened in the 1950s—ordinary people stood up for their rights and, in doing so, reshaped the course of American history. The Civil Rights Movement of this era was a beacon of hope, a courageous fight against injustice, and a testament to the power of unity and determination. Let's revisit the story of this transformative time and the incredible people who turned the tide.

The Background of Segregation

In the 1950s, segregation was still a stark reality in many parts of the United States. African Americans faced discrimination, racial prejudice, and the indignity of "separate but equal" facilities. The time was ripe for change.

The Montgomery Bus Boycott

The Civil Rights Movement of the 1950s was sparked by an act of quiet defiance that echoed across the nation. Rosa Parks, a seamstress in Montgomery, Alabama, refused to give up her seat on a city bus to a white man in December 1955. Her arrest led to a year-long boycott of the city's buses. The Montgomery Bus Boycott was a triumph of nonviolent protest and resilience.

Leaders and Visionaries

The movement was fueled by leaders and visionaries who dedicated their lives to achieving equality. Dr. Martin Luther King Jr., a Baptist minister and civil rights leader, emerged as the voice of the movement. His eloquent speeches and commitment to nonviolent protest became the heart and soul of the struggle.

Brown v. Board of Education

The landmark Supreme Court case Brown v. Board of Education in 1954 declared that racial segregation in public schools was unconstitutional. This decision was a significant victory for the Civil Rights Movement, opening the door to integration and equal educational opportunities.

Sit-Ins and Freedom Rides

In the late 1950s, "sit-ins" and "freedom rides" became powerful symbols of resistance. Young African Americans, along with sympathetic white activists, sat at segregated lunch counters and rode buses through the South to protest segregation. Their courage and commitment brought attention to the injustices they faced.

The Little Rock Nine

In 1957, nine African American students, known as the "Little Rock Nine," enrolled at Central High School in Little Rock, Arkansas. Their entrance into the formerly all-white school was met with resistance, and the federal government had to intervene to protect their right to an education.

The Civil Rights Act of 1957

In 1957, Congress passed the Civil Rights Act, the first such legislation in nearly a century. It aimed to protect the voting rights of African Americans and created a Civil Rights Division within the Department of Justice.

The Legacy of the Civil Rights Movement

The Civil Rights Movement of the 1950s laid the groundwork for the larger battles to come in the 1960s. It was a time of remarkable progress, when the determination and resilience of ordinary people led to extraordinary change. The movement demonstrated the power of nonviolent protest and the importance of unity in the face of injustice.

The legacy of the 1950s Civil Rights Movement endures today, reminding us that the fight for equality is an ongoing journey. It was a time when a few brave individuals stood up against discrimination, and their actions would inspire generations to come. The Civil Rights Movement of the 1950s was a beacon of hope and a turning point in American history, showing us that change is possible when people come together for a just and equal society.

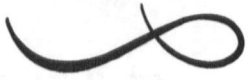

Walt's Magical Dream - Creating Disneyland

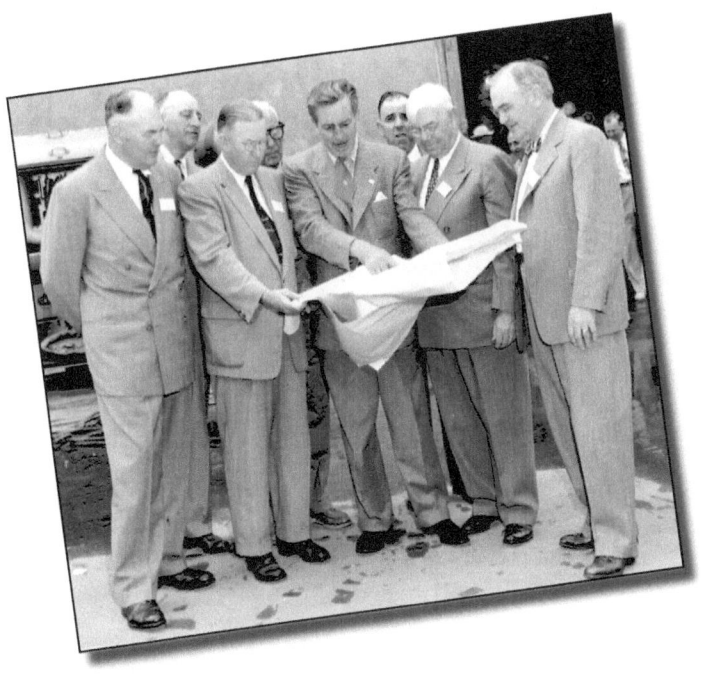

1955—the birth of Disneyland. This magical kingdom, born from the vision and determination of one of the world's most beloved storytellers, Walt Disney, would become an iconic symbol of joy, imagination, and family fun. Let's embark on a journey to discover how Disneyland came to life in the heart of 1950s America.

The Dream Takes Shape

Walt Disney had long harbored a dream of creating a place where families could escape into a world of fantasy and wonder. He envisioned a place where the enchanting tales from his films could come to life, and where people of all ages could experience joy together. The concept of Disneyland began to take shape in his imagination.

From Idea to Reality

In the early 1950s, Walt set his grand plan into motion. He wanted a theme park unlike any other—a place where dreams met reality, where imagination had no bounds. He assembled a dedicated team of artists, engineers, and designers to bring his vision to life. Together, they worked tirelessly to turn his dream into a reality.

Creating the Magic Kingdom

Disneyland wasn't just a theme park; it was a kingdom of magic, adventure, and enchantment. The park was divided into distinct lands, each with its unique theme, attractions, and stories. Main Street, Adventureland, Fantasyland, Frontierland, and Tomorrowland were the first lands to greet visitors when Disneyland opened its gates on July 17, 1955.

Opening Day and the "Disneyland" TV Special

Disneyland's opening day was a monumental event. However, it was also fraught with challenges, from scorching heat to broken rides. Yet, it was a day filled with excitement, and thousands of eager visitors flocked to the park. The event was even televised in a live broadcast called the "Disneyland" TV special, hosted by none other than Walt Disney himself.

An Instant Success

Despite some initial hiccups, Disneyland became an instant success. It enchanted visitors with iconic attractions like Sleeping Beauty Castle, the Matterhorn Bobsleds, and the Jungle Cruise. Families experienced the magic of Fantasyland, ventured into the wilds of Adventureland, and explored the possibilities of Tomorrowland.

Continual Innovation

Walt Disney was never one to rest on his laurels. He constantly sought to improve and expand the park. In 1959, Disneyland saw the introduction of the Disneyland Monorail, the Matterhorn Bobsleds, and the iconic Submarine Voyage.

A Magical Legacy

The creation of Disneyland was not just evidence of Walt Disney's creative genius; it was evidence of his unwavering belief in the power of dreams and storytelling. Disneyland became a place where young and old could escape the ordinary and journey into realms of imagination and enchantment.

It's a place where families create cherished memories, where dreams come to life, and where the magic of storytelling endures. Disneyland in the 1950s was not just an amusement park; it was a place where magic became reality, and the wonder of childhood was celebrated.

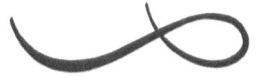

The Decade's Heroes - The Korean War

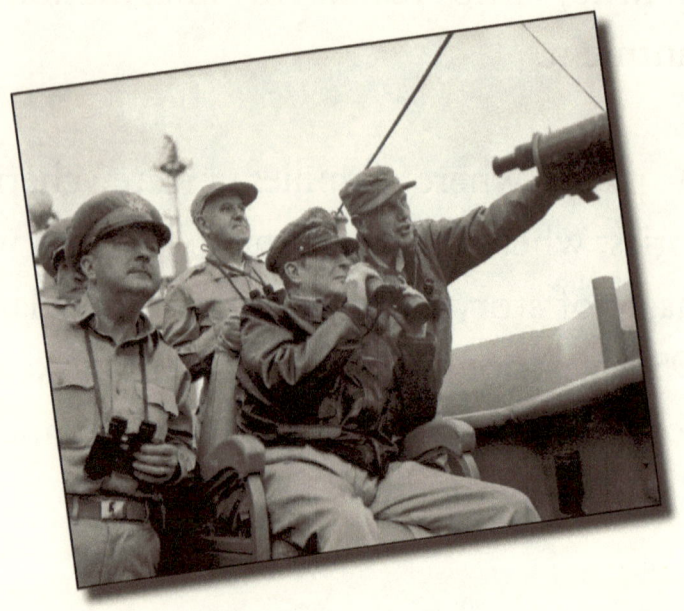

The 1950s wasn't all rock 'n' roll and smiles, it was also a time when the world was gripped by the shock and sorrow of the Korean War. The conflict in Korea holds a unique place in American history, a time when ordinary people and brave soldiers faced the challenge of defending democracy on a far-off peninsula. Let's delve into the story of the Korean War, a chapter that deserves to be remembered.

The Background of the Korean War

The Korean War, which began on June 25, 1950, was a result of the Cold War's global tensions. The Korean Peninsula had been divided at the 38th parallel into North and South Korea after World War II, with the Soviet Union supporting the North and the United States backing the South.

The Invasion and UN Response

The conflict erupted when North Korean forces, under the leadership of Kim Il-sung and with the support of the Soviet Union and China, invaded South Korea. The United Nations immediately condemned the aggression and called for collective action to defend South Korea.

The American Commitment

The United States, led by President Harry S. Truman, made a commitment to support South

Korea in the face of communist aggression. The American people, still reeling from the recent memories of World War II, rallied behind this cause to preserve democracy and freedom.

The War's Challenges

The Korean War was a challenging conflict, characterized by brutal winter conditions, mountainous terrain, and shifting battle lines. The war saw intense fighting and heavy casualties on both sides. It was also the first time that jet aircraft were used in combat, as well as the beginning of the television era, allowing people at home to witness the war's realities.

The Role of American Soldiers

American soldiers played a vital role in the Korean War. They faced extreme hardships, from freezing winters to intense combat, and displayed incredible bravery and resilience. The war was marked by the heroism of individuals like

Corporal Tibor Rubin, who was awarded the Medal of Honor for his actions as a prisoner of war.

The Armistice and Ongoing Division

The Korean War ended on July 27, 1953, with an armistice agreement, but not a formal peace treaty. The Korean Peninsula remained divided, with the North and South existing as separate nations. The war's impact on the Korean people, particularly those separated from their families, is still felt today.

Looking Back

The Korean War, often overshadowed by the larger conflicts of World War II and the Vietnam War, is sometimes referred to as the "Forgotten War." However, its legacy lives on in the dedication and sacrifice of the soldiers who fought, and in the enduring hope for peace and reunification of the Korean Peninsula.

The Korean War serves as a reminder of the price of freedom and the bravery of those who served. It was a time when the United States stood in defense of democracy and the values that make this nation great. The Korean War demonstrated the resilience and courage of those who answered the call in a distant land.

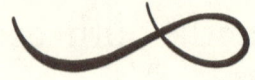

Island in Revolution - The Cuban Revolution

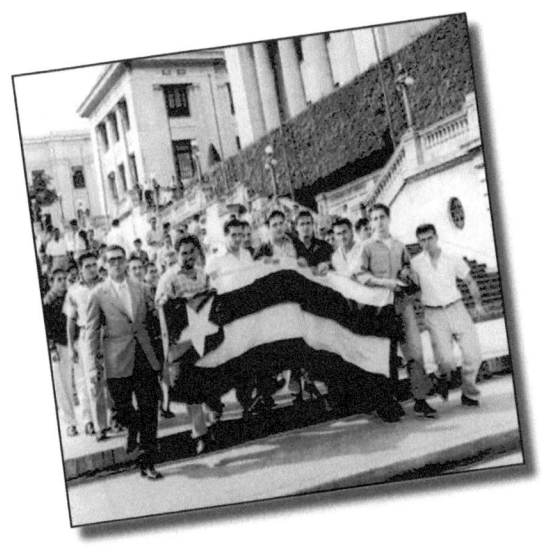

Picture this - dance parties, jukeboxes, and latin rhythms filling the air . But beneath this colorful surface, an island in the Caribbean was undergoing a profound transformation—the Cuban Revolution. This captivating story of resilience, rebellion, and change unfolded just a short distance from American shores, leaving a lasting impact on the region and the world. Join us as we delve into the turbulent times of the Cuban Revolution.

The Backdrop: Pre-Revolution Cuba

In the 1950s, Cuba was a tropical paradise known for its white sandy beaches, vibrant culture, and bustling nightlife. Tourists flocked to Havana, sipping on mojitos and dancing the night away in glamorous casinos. However, beneath this glamorous facade, a stark contrast existed.

The Rise of Fidel Castro

Enter Fidel Castro, a charismatic and determined young lawyer who became the face of the Cuban Revolution. He and a band of rebels, including the iconic Che Guevara, waged a guerrilla war against the dictatorship of Fulgencio Batista. Their message of justice, equality, and an end to corruption resonated with many Cubans.

The Revolutionary Struggle

For years, the rebels fought from the Sierra Maestra mountains, gaining support and momentum. As their cause grew, they garnered international attention and sympathy, particularly from those who believed in their mission to topple a corrupt regime and improve the lives of ordinary Cubans.

The Fall of Batista

On January 1, 1959, Batista fled the country, marking the culmination of the Cuban Revolution. The people of Cuba celebrated in the streets, believing that a new era of justice and prosperity was dawning.

The United States and the Revolution

The Cuban Revolution created a complicated relationship between the United States and the new Cuban government. Initially, the U.S. extended diplomatic recognition to Castro's government, but as the revolution took a more socialist turn and nationalized American-owned businesses, tensions escalated.

The Bay of Pigs and the Cuban Missile Crisis

In the early 1960s, the Bay of Pigs invasion, a failed CIA-led operation, strained relations between the U.S. and Cuba. This was followed by the Cuban Missile Crisis, a tense standoff between the U.S. and the Soviet Union on Cuban soil. The crisis had the world on the brink of nuclear war before a peaceful resolution was reached.

The Impact of the Revolution

The Cuban Revolution brought about significant changes in Cuba, including land reforms, improvements in education and healthcare, and efforts to address issues of inequality. However, it also led to political repression, a one-party system, and a state-controlled economy.

The Cuban Revolution was a turning point in the history of the Americas.. Though the revolution's legacy is still a subject of debate, its impact on the course of history cannot be denied.

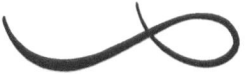

Bridges and Barricades - Hungary and Suez

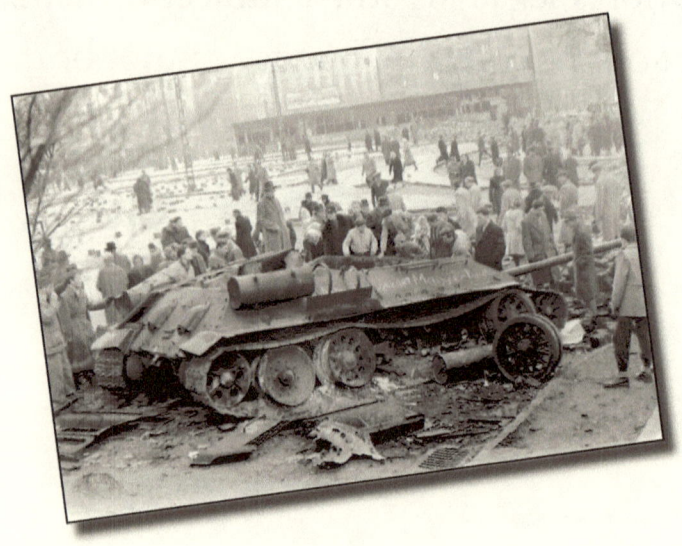

The 1950s were a time of international intrigue and political high-stakes, with the world's superpowers, the United States and the Soviet Union, jockeying for influence on the global stage. Two events, the Hungarian Revolution and the Suez Crisis, emerged as pivotal moments in this Cold War era. They showcased the intricate dance of power, ideology, and diplomacy that characterized this remarkable period. Let's explore these two concurrent crises and the superpower standoff that unfolded in the United States.

The Hungarian Revolution of 1956

In the autumn of 1956, the world watched in awe as the Hungarian people rose up against their Soviet-controlled government. Hungary had been under Soviet influence since the end of World War II, and the people's frustration with their communist regime had reached a boiling point.

The Spark of Revolt

The revolution began as a student protest but quickly spread to encompass a wide range of societal groups. Hungarian citizens took to the streets, demanding political reform, freedom, and an end to Soviet control.

The World Watches

News of the Hungarian Revolution resonated worldwide, including in the United States. Americans sympathized with the Hungarians' yearning for freedom and cheered on their fight for self-determination.

Soviet Intervention

However, the United States and the world watched in shock as Soviet forces invaded Hungary in late 1956 to suppress the rebellion. The superpower standoff became apparent as the U.S. grappled with the challenge of how to respond to Soviet aggression without sparking a larger conflict.

Suez Crisis of 1956

Simultaneously, another crisis was unfolding in the Middle East—the Suez Crisis. Egypt's President Gamal Abdel Nasser nationalized the

Suez Canal, a crucial waterway controlled by British and French companies. This move threatened their access to vital oil supplies.

Differing Responses

The United States, under President Dwight D. Eisenhower, and the Soviet Union, led by Premier Nikita Khrushchev, both sought to exert influence during the Suez Crisis. The superpowers' differing responses revealed the complexity of the era.

Eisenhower Doctrine and Pressure

President Eisenhower, fearing that military action might escalate the Cold War, pressured Britain, France, and Israel to withdraw their forces from the Suez Canal. He also introduced the Eisenhower Doctrine, offering U.S. assistance to countries resisting communism.

End of the Crises

The Hungarian Revolution ended in tragedy as Soviet forces brutally suppressed the uprising, leaving a deep scar on the Hungarian people. Meanwhile, the Suez Crisis resulted in a U.S.-led resolution that led to the withdrawal of foreign troops from the Suez Canal.

The Superpower Standoff

The Hungarian Revolution and the Suez Crisis were emblematic of the superpower standoff of the 1950s. The United States and the Soviet Union grappled for influence, with both crises highlighting the complexities of the Cold War era.

These events are a reminder of a world teetering on the brink, where the choices of a few leaders could have far-reaching consequences for nations and people around the globe. A time when the world held its breath and the United States, as a global leader, played a pivotal role in shaping the course of history.

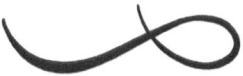

Shaking Up the Nation - The Birth of Rock 'n' Roll

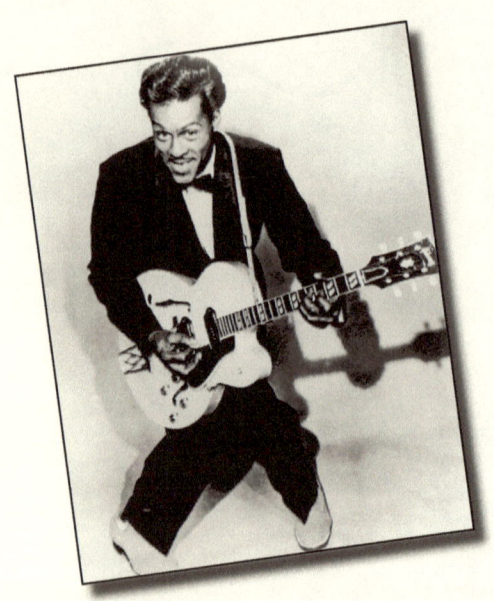

The 1950s were a time of cultural transformation in America, and at the heart of this revolution was the birth of rock 'n' roll. Two names, Elvis Presley and Chuck Berry, stand out as the architects of a new musical era that would sweep the nation and change the course of music history. Let's turn up the volume and imagine the sound of the electric guitar as we explore the incredible impact of these two musical legends.

Elvis Presley: The King of Rock 'n' Roll

In the mid-1950s, a young, charismatic Elvis Presley burst onto the music scene with a sound and style that would captivate the nation. Born in Tupelo, Mississippi, and later making his home in Memphis, Tennessee, Elvis embodied the fusion of blues, gospel, and country that defined rock 'n' roll.

The Sun Sessions

Elvis began his meteoric rise in 1954 when he recorded a string of songs at Sun Studio, including "That's All Right" and "Blue Moon of Kentucky." His raw energy and undeniable charisma ignited a sensation that hadn't been seen before.

Elvis on Television

Elvis's appearance on national television, particularly his scandalous hip-shaking on "The

Ed Sullivan Show," solidified his status as a cultural icon. He became the voice of a generation, and his legions of fans, known as "Elvis Presley's Army," carried the rock 'n' roll torch with pride.

Chuck Berry: The Father of Rock 'n' Roll Guitar

Meanwhile, in St. Louis, Missouri, Chuck Berry was crafting his own brand of rock 'n' roll. With his distinctive guitar playing, witty lyrics, and captivating stage presence, he became a true pioneer of the genre.

"Maybellene" and "Johnny B. Goode"

In 1955, Chuck Berry released "Maybellene," a groundbreaking hit that fused elements of blues, country, and rhythm and blues into a distinctive rock 'n' roll sound. He followed it up with classics like "Roll Over Beethoven" and "Johnny B. Goode," which are still celebrated today.

Breaking Racial Barriers

Both Elvis and Chuck Berry challenged racial barriers by introducing black music to white audiences. Their music brought people together on the dance floor and helped bridge gaps in a segregated society.

Rock 'n' Roll's Impact

The emergence of rock 'n' roll had a profound impact on American culture. It provided an outlet for self-expression, youthful rebellion, and a shared experience. Teens across the country embraced the music and its accompanying dance styles, from the jitterbug to the twist.

The Lasting Impact of Elvis and Chuck Berry

Elvis and Chuck Berry left an indelible mark on music and culture. Their influence can be heard in the work of countless artists who followed in their footsteps, from The Beatles to Bruce Springsteen. Their songs continue to be celebrated, covered, and cherished by new generations of music lovers.

A Musical Revolution

The 1950s marked a musical revolution, led by the likes of Elvis Presley and Chuck Berry. Their pioneering spirit and innovative sound created a new genre that would shape the future of music. In this vibrant era of social change and cultural exploration, rock 'n' roll emerged as the soundtrack of a generation, uniting young and old, black and white, and leaving an indelible groove on the American soul. So, let's put on our blue suede shoes, twist again like we did last summer, and thank the pioneers who made rock 'n' roll a force to be reckoned with.

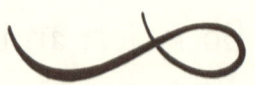

Changing Channels - Television and Culture

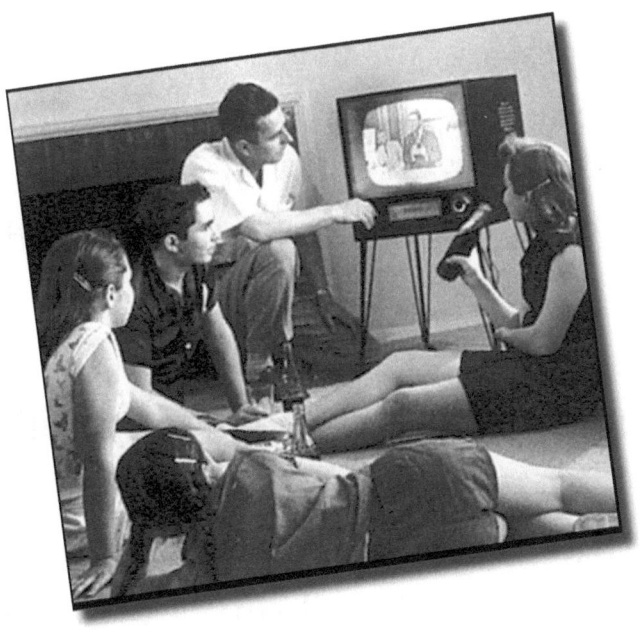

Don't be a square, something exciting is on the flickering screens of television sets. Television emerges as a central figure in the lives of millions, influencing everything from fashion to family dynamics. Let's channel hop to this golden era of television and its profound impact on popular culture.

The Birth of the TV Age

In the post-World War II years, television sets began appearing in living rooms across the country. Families gathered around to watch the likes of "I Love Lucy," "The Honeymooners," and "The Ed Sullivan Show" on their black-and-white screens.

Lucille Ball: The Queen of Comedy

Lucille Ball became a household name with her iconic role as Lucy Ricardo in "I Love Lucy." Her zany antics, hilarious mishaps, and unwavering charm made her America's favorite redhead and a trailblazing figure for women in the entertainment industry.

Sullivan's Showcase

"The Ed Sullivan Show" was a variety program that featured a diverse range of acts, from Elvis Presley's electrifying performances to the astonishing talents of The Beatles. Sullivan's show was a cultural touchstone, introducing the nation to the latest trends in music, comedy, and dance.

The American Dream on Display

Television showcased the American Dream in many forms. In "Leave It to Beaver," we saw the wholesome Cleaver family, reflecting an idealized suburban life. "Father Knows Best" and "The Donna Reed Show" reinforced traditional family values.

Television Redefined Fashion

TV stars of the 1950s became style icons. Marilyn Monroe's sultry looks influenced fashion, and James Dean's rebel style was emulated by teenagers. The "poodle skirt" and the "greaser" look were just a few examples of how television shaped clothing choices.

The Twilight Zone:
A Journey into the Unknown

Not all television of the '50s was lighthearted. "The Twilight Zone," created by Rod Serling, delved into the mysterious, the bizarre, and the thought-provoking. It challenged viewers to question the status quo and explore the realms of the unknown.

Television and Civil Rights

Television played a pivotal role in bringing the Civil Rights Movement to the forefront of American consciousness. News coverage and programs like "The Nat King Cole Show" offered a platform for African American voices and inspired social change.

The Power of Advertising

Television introduced a powerful new medium for advertising. Iconic jingles like "I'd Like to Buy the World a Coke" and memorable ad campaigns created an indelible connection between brands and consumers.

The Advent of Color Television

In the late 1950s, color television made its debut, changing the way some viewers experienced their favorite shows. Color sets became coveted possessions, and advertisers made the most of this new dimension, but most Americans had black and white television until the next decade.

Television Today

The 1950s brought us the magic of television, turning living rooms into theaters and transforming the way we connected with each other and the world. Television in the '50s was more than a screen; it was a window into our hopes, dreams, and shared experiences.

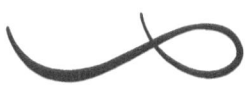

The Glory Days - Sports in 1950s America

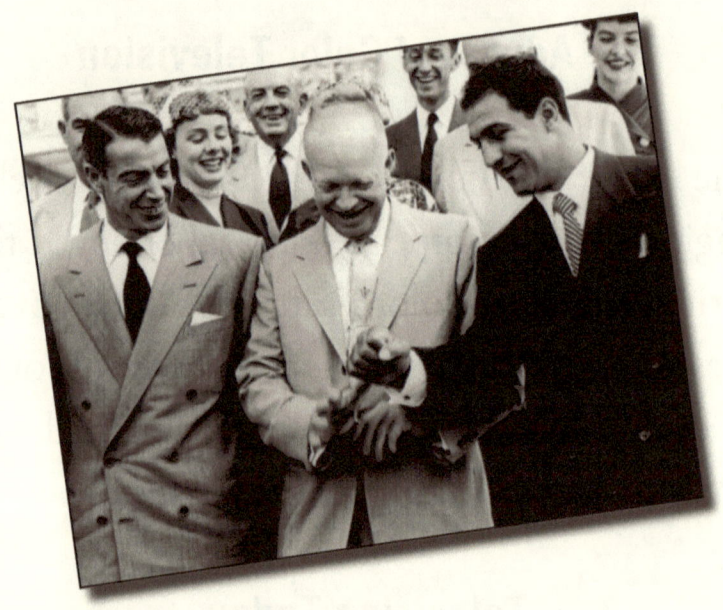

Let's step into our time machine and journey back to the 1950s, an era filled with dazzling athleticism, legendary athletes, and unforgettable sporting moments. The '50s were a time when sports took center stage in American culture, providing excitement, inspiration, and a sense of unity. In this article, we'll explore the vibrant world of sports during this remarkable decade.

Baseball: The National Pastime

In the 1950s, baseball reigned as the undisputed "national pastime." Iconic players like Mickey Mantle, Willie Mays, and Ted Williams graced the diamond, capturing the hearts of fans across the country. The New York Yankees dominated the era, winning numerous championships and solidifying their place in baseball history.

The Birth of Modern Football

The 1950s saw the NFL transform from a fledgling league into a major sporting powerhouse. Legends like Johnny Unitas, Jim Brown, and Bart Starr made their mark on the gridiron, shaping the future of American football.

Magical Moments in Boxing

The world of boxing witnessed some of its most iconic bouts in the 1950s. The rivalry between Rocky Marciano and Jersey Joe Walcott, Sugar Ray Robinson's graceful boxing style, and the emergence of a young Cassius Clay (who would later become Muhammad Ali) captivated fight fans around the globe.

The Heart-Pounding Drama of College Basketball

College basketball hit its stride in the '50s, with fierce rivalries and epic showdowns becoming an integral part of the American sports landscape. The University of Kentucky, coached by Adolph Rupp, and the University of Kansas, led by Phog Allen, were among the dominant teams of the decade.

The Olympics: A Platform for Heroes

The 1950s marked the return of the Olympics after a 12-year hiatus due to World War II. The first post-war Summer Olympics took place in 1952 in Helsinki, Finland. The Games provided a stage for sporting heroes like Wilma Rudolph, who overcame adversity to become the "fastest woman in the world," and the unforgettable performance of Roger Bannister, who ran the first sub-four-minute mile.

Women in Sports: A New Frontier

The 1950s were also a time of progress for women in sports. Icons like Althea Gibson shattered racial barriers in tennis, while Babe Didrikson Zaharias proved that women could excel in multiple sports, from golf to track and field.

The Dynamic Duo: The Harlem Globetrotters

The Harlem Globetrotters dazzled audiences with their basketball wizardry and comedic antics. They transcended racial and cultural barriers, becoming international ambassadors of goodwill.

Sports on Television

Television brought the thrill of sports into American living rooms. Game of the Week broadcasts in baseball and NFL games on Sundays became cherished traditions. Television made sports accessible to a wider audience and elevated athletes to celebrity status.

The Heart of the American Spirit

Sports in the 1950s reflected the heart of the American spirit—determination, teamwork, and the pursuit of excellence. It was a time when sports served as a unifying force, bringing people together to cheer for their favorite teams and athletes.

The 1950s were a golden era in American sports, filled with legendary figures, unforgettable moments, and a sense of camaraderie that transcended the playing field. These sports icons and moments continue to hold a special place in the hearts of sports enthusiasts and serve as a reminder of the enduring power of athletic achievement. The '50s were a time when the nation cheered for its heroes, and sports, in all its glory, offered a collective sense of pride and inspiration.

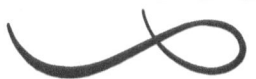

Celebrating Champions - Sporting Results

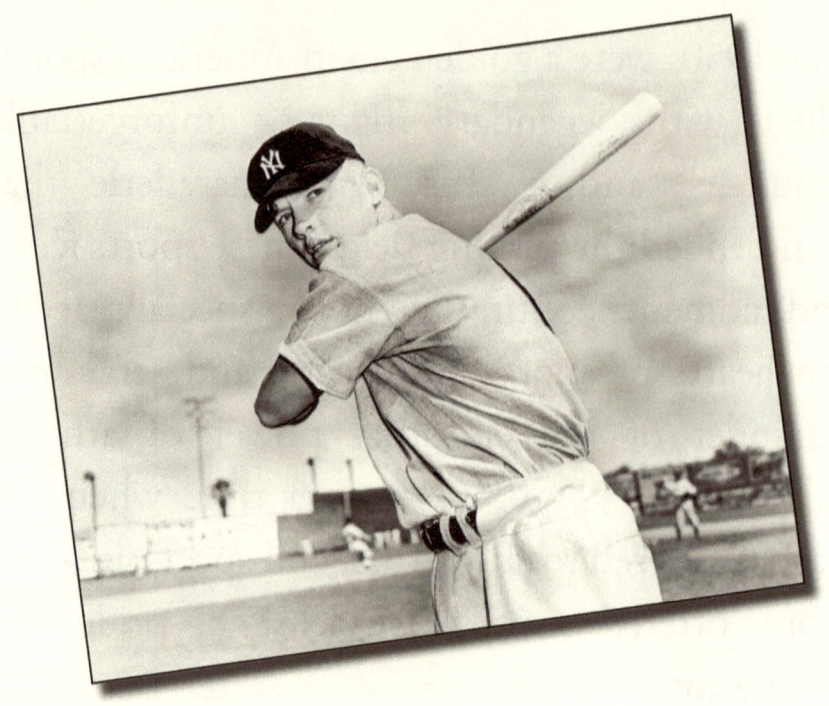

The 1950s were a decade of sporting triumphs, where legends were made, records shattered, and memories etched into the annals of American sports history. From the baseball diamonds to the boxing rings, this article is a friendly reminder of the remarkable sporting results that enthralled the nation during this dynamic era.

Baseball's Yankee Dynasty

The New York Yankees were the undisputed kings of baseball in the 1950s. With legendary figures like Mickey Mantle, Yogi Berra, and Whitey Ford, they clinched multiple World Series titles, securing their place in baseball lore. The 1950 World Series saw the Yankees victorious over the Philadelphia Phillies, and they continued their dominance with wins in 1951, 1952, 1953, 1956, and 1958. The Yankees' unparalleled success defined the decade's baseball scene.

The Miracle of the Giants

The New York Giants' dramatic victory over the Brooklyn Dodgers in the 1951 National League playoff, often referred to as the "Shot Heard 'Round the World" (Bobby Thomson's home run), remains one of the most famous moments in baseball history.

Rise of Rocky Marciano

In the realm of boxing, Rocky Marciano emerged as a formidable force. In 1952, he defeated Jersey Joe Walcott to become the heavyweight champion of the world, a title he successfully defended until his retirement in 1956. His unblemished record of 49 wins, including 43 by knockout, remains the stuff of boxing legends.

Jim Brown's Gridiron Greatness

Jim Brown, one of the most dominant players in the history of the National Football League (NFL), burst onto the scene in the 1950s. He led the league in rushing yards for eight consecutive seasons and set numerous records. His remarkable achievements with the Cleveland Browns left an indelible mark on football history.

The Perfect Season:
The 1957-58 Boston Celtics

The Boston Celtics, led by Bill Russell and coach Red Auerbach, completed one of the most remarkable seasons in NBA history. They went on to win the NBA championship with a perfect postseason record, a feat that has been rarely equaled in professional basketball.

The Heart of Sportsmanship:
Willie Mays and "The Catch"

Willie Mays, the "Say Hey Kid," delivered a spectacular moment in the 1954 World Series. Playing center field for the New York Giants, Mays made an over-the-shoulder, basket-style catch, widely known as "The Catch," which is still celebrated as one of the greatest plays in baseball history.

Olympic Triumphs and Athletic Achievements

The 1950s were a decade of Olympic excellence. Athletes like Wilma Rudolph, who overcame adversity to win three gold medals in track and field at the 1960 Summer Olympics, and Bob Mathias, who became the first person to win back-to-back decathlon golds, inspired the nation with their exceptional performances.

Wimbledon Wonders: Althea Gibson

Althea Gibson made history in 1957 by becoming the first African American to win a Grand Slam title at Wimbledon. Her victory in women's singles and doubles marked a milestone in the sport and shattered racial barriers.

The 1950s were a time of sporting heroes, historic achievements, and unforgettable moments. From the baseball diamond to the boxing ring, the football field, and the Olympic podium, athletes displayed unwavering dedication and passion for their sports, leaving an enduring legacy in the hearts of fans. These sporting results remind us of the magic that happens when athletes push the boundaries of human potential and unite a nation through the love of the game.

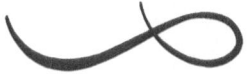

Feasting on Nostalgia - Food in 1950s America

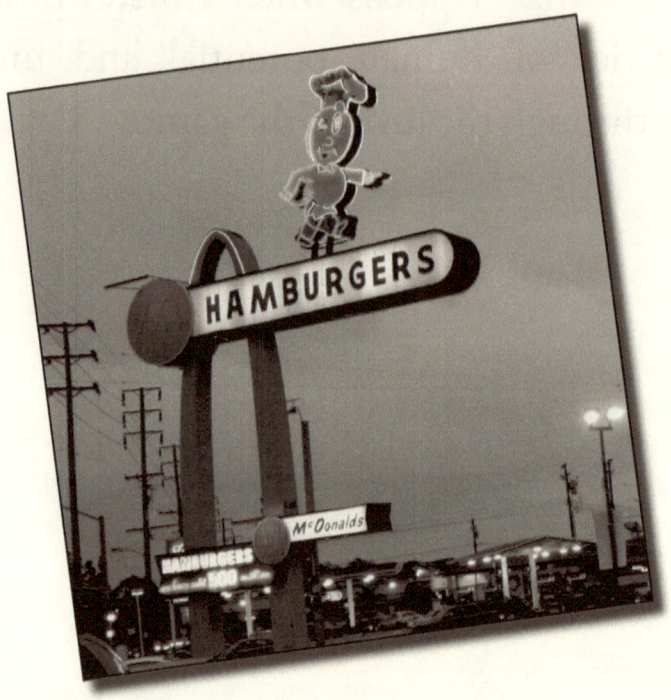

Let's step into the charming world of the 1950s, a time when dining tables were adorned with classic comfort foods, soda fountains served up fizzy delights, and family recipes were treasured like gold. In this article, we'll take a friendly stroll down memory lane and revisit the delectable flavors and culinary trends that defined food in 1950s America.

The Rise of Convenience Foods

The 1950s marked the birth of convenience foods. Products like TV dinners and canned soups promised to simplify meal preparation for busy families. The concept of frozen, pre-packaged meals was revolutionary, giving homemakers a break in the kitchen.

The All-American Burger

The hamburger became a symbol of American fast food culture in the 1950s. Iconic burger joints like McDonald's and Burger King made their debut, offering up delicious, no-fuss fare that catered to the on-the-go lifestyle of the era.

Soda Fountains and Milkshakes

Soda fountains were a cherished part of the '50s dining experience. These establishments served up classic soda flavors, malted milkshakes, and indulgent ice cream sundaes, creating cherished memories of shared treats and sweet nostalgia.

Jell-O Everything

Jell-O, the wobbly dessert, was a staple in 1950s households. From salads to molded desserts, Jell-O's versatility and vibrant colors made it a creative culinary canvas for home cooks.

TV Dinners: A Taste of Modernity

TV dinners, introduced in 1953, revolutionized mealtime. These pre-packaged trays contained a mix of meat, vegetables, and dessert, providing a convenient way for families to dine while watching their favorite shows.

The Casserole Craze

Casserole dishes, often laden with creamed soups and cheese, became a popular choice for homemakers in the '50s. They offered an easy and economical way to feed a family, and many recipes became treasured heirlooms.

Classic Comfort Foods

Potato salad, meatloaf, macaroni and cheese, and deviled eggs were classic comfort foods that graced American tables. These dishes were a testament to the warmth and simplicity of home-cooked meals.

Moms as Culinary Queens

The 1950s celebrated the image of the quintessential homemaker and her culinary prowess. Women were seen as the family's culinary queens, creating nourishing and flavorful meals that brought families together.

The Can-Opener Chef

Canned goods played a prominent role in 1950s cooking. Canned vegetables, soups, and fruits found their way into many dishes, adding convenience and flavor.

The Cocktail Hour

Cocktail parties were a hallmark of the era. Classic concoctions like the Martini, Old Fashioned, and Manhattan took center stage at social gatherings, accompanied by elegant appetizers and snacks.

Diner Delights

Diners and drive-ins were the go-to spots for late-night meals and weekend excursions. Here, you could savor juicy burgers, crispy fries, and creamy milkshakes, creating memories that have stood the test of time.

The food of the 1950s was a reflection of an era that celebrated simplicity, convenience, and the comforts of home. From TV dinners to classic American diners, it was a time of culinary innovation and traditions passed down through generations. The flavors of the '50s continue to hold a special place in the hearts and palates of those who grew up savoring the delicious tastes of a bygone era. It's a reminder that the joy of good food and shared meals transcends time and trends.

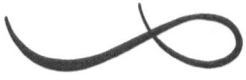

On the Road Again -
The Wheels of Change

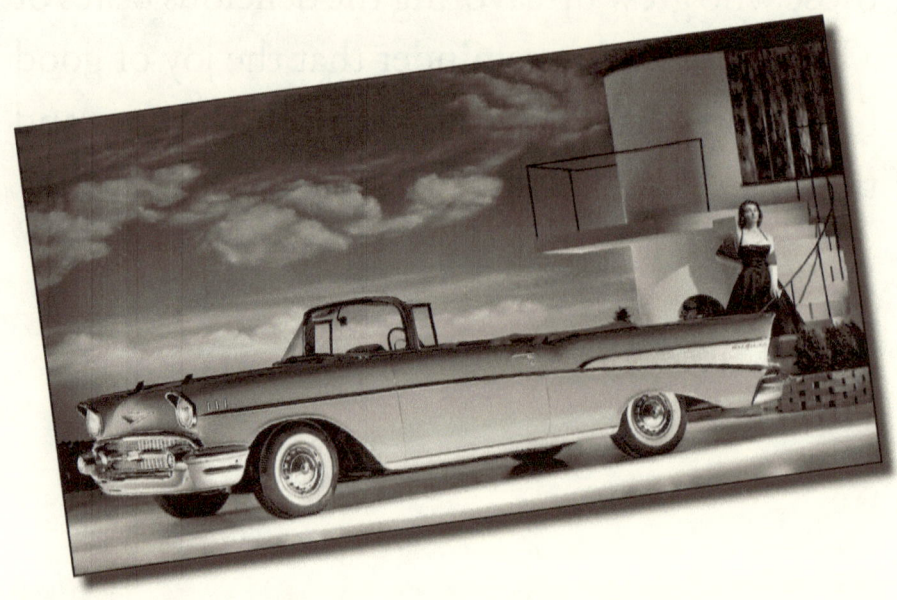

Want to journey back to the open roads and the spirit of adventure that defined 1950s America? This was a time when the automobile was king, the skies belonged to jet planes, and trains crisscrossed the nation, making travel more accessible than ever. In this article, we'll explore the fascinating world of transportation in the '50s and how it shaped the way Americans moved, connected, and explored.

The Automobile Revolution

The 1950s marked the peak of the American love affair with the automobile. It was the decade of chrome and tailfins, when cars weren't just a mode of transportation but a symbol of style and status.

Drive-Ins and Drive-Thrus

The era of car culture brought us drive-in theaters, where families and young couples could catch the latest movies without leaving their cars. And let's not forget the drive-thru, a convenient innovation that changed the way we ordered food and coffee.

The Interstate Highway System

One of the most significant transportation achievements of the 1950s was the development of the Interstate Highway System. Signed into law by President Dwight D. Eisenhower in 1956, this massive infrastructure project revolutionized travel, connecting cities and states and making long-distance road trips easier and more efficient.

Iconic American Cars

The '50s introduced us to iconic automobiles like the Chevrolet Bel Air, the Ford Thunderbird, and the Cadillac Eldorado. These cars represented freedom, mobility, and the American dream.

Travel by Air: The Jet Age Takes Off

The advent of jet travel in the 1950s brought a new level of speed and excitement to air travel. The Boeing 707, known as the "Jet Clipper," became the first commercially successful jetliner, making transcontinental and international travel faster and more accessible.

The Golden Age of Trains

While air travel was on the rise, trains still played a significant role in American transportation. The 1950s were considered the golden age of rail travel, with luxurious trains like the Super Chief and the 20th Century Limited offering passengers an elegant and comfortable journey.

Greyhound Buses: Rolling Across America

Greyhound buses provided an essential mode of transportation for those who preferred the open road but didn't want to drive. The recognizable silver buses crisscrossed the nation, connecting cities and towns.

Transporting Goods:
The Rise of the Trucking Industry

The 1950s saw the expansion of the trucking industry, which played a crucial role in transporting goods and supplies across the country. The modernization of trucking systems and infrastructure revolutionized logistics and distribution.

Traveling in Style: Airstream Trailers

The Airstream trailer, with its iconic, streamlined design, offered a new way to travel and explore America's vast landscapes. These stylish trailers became symbols of adventure and wanderlust.

The Family Road Trip: An American Tradition

The 1950s cemented the family road trip as an American tradition. Families packed up their cars and hit the highway to explore the nation's national parks, historic landmarks, and scenic byways.

Transportation in 1950s America was about more than just getting from point A to point B. It was about freedom, adventure, and the pursuit of the American dream. Whether it was cruising down Route 66 in a classic convertible or embarking on a cross-country train journey, the '50s were a time of exploration and excitement on the open road and in the skies. These modes of transport weren't just vehicles; they were the vessels of dreams and memories, connecting people to the vast and diverse landscapes of America.

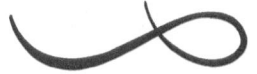

Glamour and Grace - Fashion in 1950s America

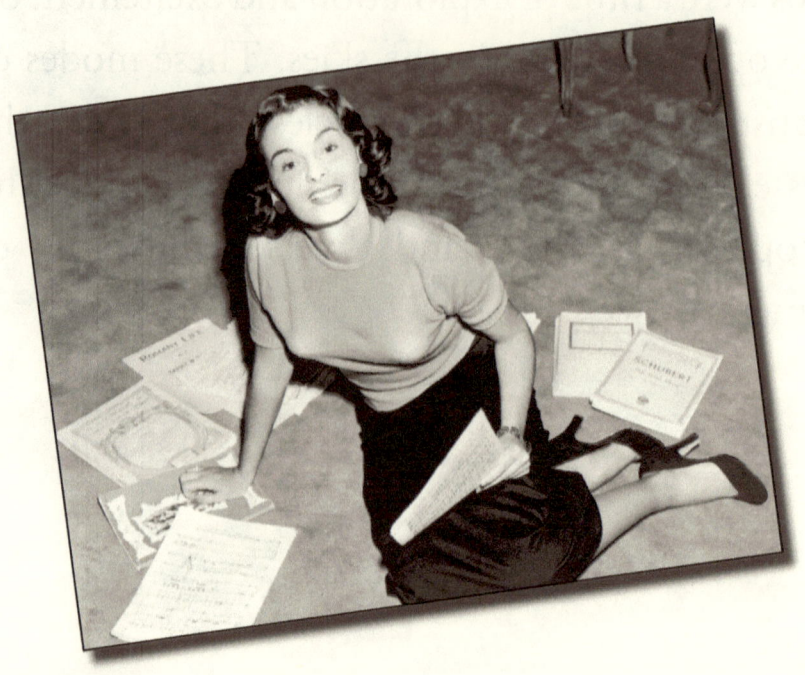

Let's dress up as we take a trip down memory lane to the decade that epitomized glamour, elegance, and the birth of iconic fashion trends. The '50s brought a renaissance in style, with men and women embracing classic looks and making fashion a form of self-expression. In this article, we'll explore the enchanting world of fashion in 1950s America.

The New Look: Christian Dior's Influence

The decade began with the lingering influence of Christian Dior's "New Look" from the late 1940s. This style was characterized by cinched waists, full skirts, and an overall emphasis on a woman's hourglass figure. The '50s marked the height of this silhouette.

The Hourglass Figure: Iconic Women's Fashion

Women's fashion in the '50s was all about accentuating the curves. Full skirts with petticoats, cinched waists, and fitted bodices were the norm. The classic shirtwaist dress, often adorned with a belt, was a wardrobe staple.

Poodle Skirts and Circle Skirts

The poodle skirt, with its playful motifs and voluminous shape, became an emblematic fashion piece. Circle skirts were equally popular, offering a twirl-worthy elegance that was perfect for dancing.

The Influence of Hollywood Stars

Hollywood played a significant role in fashion. Style icons like Audrey Hepburn, Grace Kelly, and Marilyn Monroe inspired women's fashion. Audrey's chic and simple elegance, Grace's timeless grace, and Marilyn's sultry allure left an indelible mark.

Men's Suits: The Suave Gentlemen

Men's fashion was all about sharp dressing. The classic suit was a staple in every man's closet. Tailored, well-fitted suits were the order of the day, often accompanied by a skinny tie and fedora hat.

Leather Jackets and Rebel Style

The 1950s also saw the rise of leather jackets, which became an emblem of rebellion, as popularized by figures like James Dean in "Rebel Without a Cause." The look was all about cool, casual sophistication.

Teen Fashion:
Paving the Way for Rock 'n' Roll

Teenagers embraced their own unique style, marking the birth of youth fashion. Poodle skirts, saddle shoes, and letterman jackets were all the rage, setting the stage for the rock 'n' roll revolution of the late '50s.

Accessories and Glamour

The 1950s were not just about clothing; accessories played a vital role in fashion. From pearls to cat-eye glasses, gloves to clutch purses, these accents added an extra layer of glamour and sophistication.

Hairstyles: The Beauty of Elegance

Hairstyles in the '50s were as iconic as the fashion. Women often sported classic updos, like the French twist and the beehive. Men adopted sleek, slicked-back looks, completing their dapper ensembles.

The Housewife Look:
The Perfect Homemaker

The image of the "perfect" housewife was prevalent in the '50s, and her fashion reflected it. Flouncy dresses, pearls, and neatly styled hair were considered the epitome of the era's feminine ideal.

The 1950s were a time of glamour and grace, with fashion as a form of self-expression. From the polished look of the Hollywood stars to the rebellious allure of leather jackets, the decade offered a rich tapestry of styles. These iconic fashion trends continue to inspire and captivate, proving that the elegance and charm of the '50s never go out of style. It's a reminder that fashion is not just about clothing; it's about expressing individuality and embracing the beauty of every era.

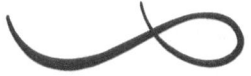

Pioneering Progress - Inventions and Science

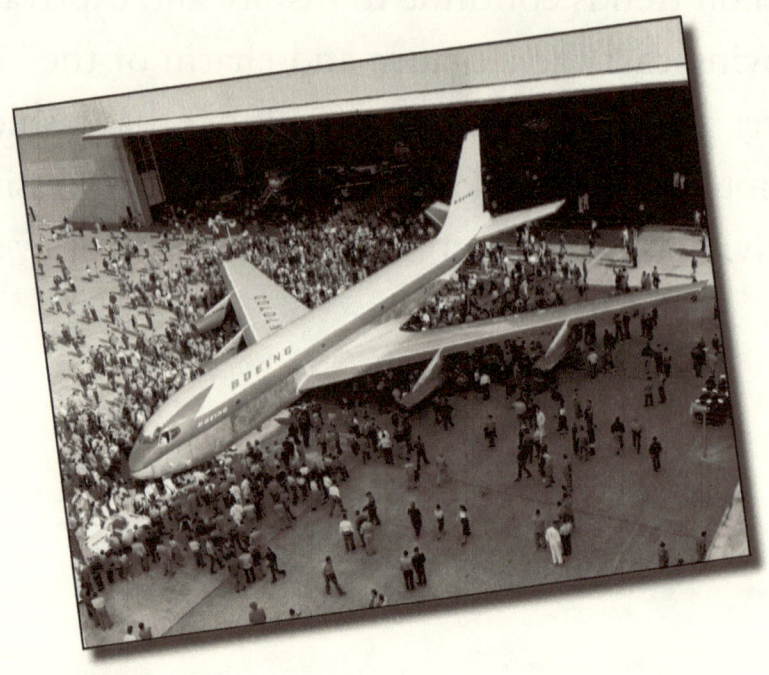

The 1950s in America was a time of immense technological advancement and scientific discovery. From the space race to groundbreaking inventions, this was a decade that laid the foundation for the future. In this article, we'll explore the pioneering progress of inventions and science innovations that shaped the '50s and beyond.

The Birth of the Transistor

One of the most significant breakthroughs of the 1950s was the invention of the transistor. This tiny but revolutionary electronic component marked the beginning of the digital age. Transistors made electronics smaller, more efficient, and led to the development of the microchip, a cornerstone of modern technology.

Television in Color

The 1950s saw the development of color television. This innovation transformed the way we experienced visual media, introducing vibrant, lifelike colors to our screens. It marked a new era in entertainment and paved the way for today's high-definition displays.

The Polio Vaccine: A Lifesaver

Dr. Jonas Salk's development of the polio vaccine in 1955 was a medical triumph. It not only saved countless lives but also marked a turning point in the fight against infectious diseases. The vaccine's success demonstrated the power of scientific research and immunization programs.

The Birth of Silicon Valley

The '50s laid the groundwork for what would become Silicon Valley. The region's emergence as a hub for innovation, technology, and entrepreneurship can be traced back to this era, with pioneering companies like Fairchild Semiconductor and Hewlett-Packard starting their journeys.

The Space Age Begins

The Cold War fueled the space race, and the 1950s marked the start of America's journey into space. In 1957, the Soviet Union launched Sputnik, the world's first artificial satellite. In response, the United States founded NASA in 1958, with the goal of exploring outer space. The

1950s laid the foundation for the Apollo program and the historic moon landing in 1969.

The First Commercial Jetliner

The Boeing 707, introduced in 1958, marked a turning point in commercial aviation. It was the first commercially successful jetliner, making air travel faster and more accessible. This innovation transformed the airline industry and brought distant destinations closer to home.

The Creation of the Credit Card

The first universal credit card, the Diners Club Card, was introduced in 1950. It revolutionized how people made purchases and carried out financial transactions, shaping modern consumer culture.

The Birth of the Barbie Doll

In 1959, the iconic Barbie doll was introduced by Mattel. This innovation transformed the toy industry, offering a new level of creative play for children and marking the beginning of a beloved cultural icon.

The Microwave Oven: A Culinary Revolution

The 1950s brought us the commercial microwave oven. Although it was initially large and expensive, it heralded a new era of convenience and revolutionized the way we cooked and reheated food.

The 1950s were a remarkable decade of scientific innovation and technological progress. These breakthroughs not only transformed our daily lives but also shaped the course of history. The spirit of discovery and the drive for innovation that defined the '50s continue to inspire today's scientists, engineers, and inventors. This era reminds us that with ingenuity, determination, and a vision for a better future, anything is possible.

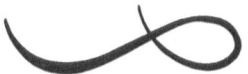

Hollywood's Golden Era - Famous Actors

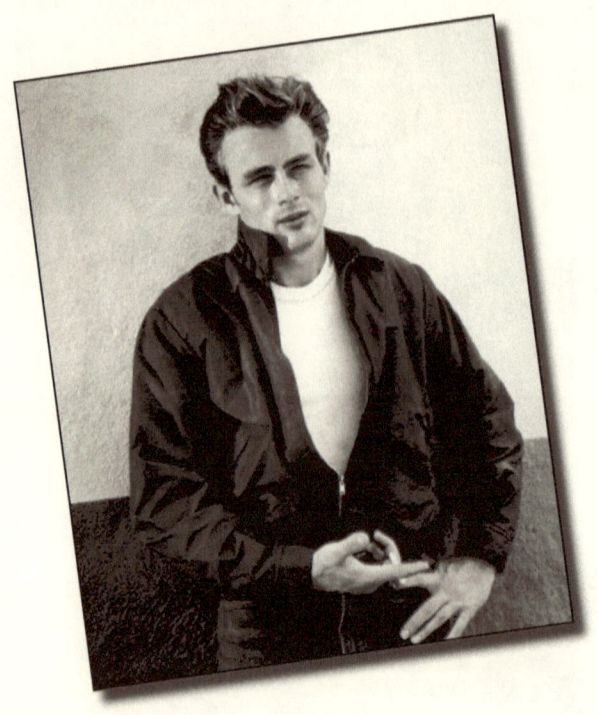

The 1950s were a magical time for American cinema, with Hollywood's golden era in full swing. It was a period of cinematic legends, where the silver screen sparkled with talent, charisma, and unforgettable performances. In this article, we'll take a friendly stroll down the red carpet and revisit the iconic actors and actresses who graced the screens of the '50s.

Marilyn Monroe:
The Ultimate Hollywood Icon

Marilyn Monroe remains the quintessential symbol of beauty and glamour. Her sensuality and charismatic presence on screen made her an enduring legend. Films like "Some Like It Hot" and "The Seven Year Itch" showcased her comedic talent, while "Gentlemen Prefer Blondes" and "Niagara" highlighted her stunning beauty.

James Dean: Rebel With a Cause

James Dean's short but impactful career left an indelible mark. His roles in "Rebel Without a Cause," "East of Eden," and "Giant" made him a symbol of youthful rebellion and vulnerability. Dean's untimely death in 1955 only added to his mystique and legend.

Audrey Hepburn: Elegance Personified

Audrey Hepburn epitomized grace and sophistication. Her roles in "Breakfast at Tiffany's," "Roman Holiday," and "Sabrina" showcased her charm and impeccable style. She became an icon of timeless elegance and humanitarianism.

Cary Grant: The Epitome of Suave

Cary Grant was the embodiment of suavity. His leading roles in films like "North by Northwest," "To Catch a Thief," and "An Affair to Remember" made him the ultimate leading man of the era. His charismatic performances continue to charm audiences today.

Grace Kelly: From Hollywood to Royalty

Grace Kelly's transition from Hollywood actress to Princess of Monaco captured the world's imagination. Her performances in films like "Rear Window," "To Catch a Thief," and "High

Noon" showcased her beauty and talent. Her real-life fairy tale added to her allure.

Marlon Brando: Method Acting Pioneer

Marlon Brando was a pioneer of method acting, bringing realism to the screen. His performances in "A Streetcar Named Desire," "On the Waterfront," and "The Wild One" transformed the art of acting and left a profound impact on the industry.

Elizabeth Taylor: A Star From Childhood

Elizabeth Taylor was a child star who transitioned into a legendary actress. Her roles in films like "Cleopatra," "Cat on a Hot Tin Roof," and "Who's Afraid of Virginia Woolf?" earned her Oscars and cemented her status as a Hollywood icon.

Paul Newman: The Blue-Eyed Charmer

Paul Newman's piercing blue eyes and rugged charm made him an icon of '50s and '60s cinema. His roles in "Cool Hand Luke," "Cat on a Hot Tin Roof," and "The Hustler" showcased his versatility and charisma.

Doris Day: America's Sweetheart

Doris Day was America's sweetheart, known for her wholesome image and delightful performances in films like "Pillow Talk," "Calamity Jane," and "The Man Who Knew Too Much." She was a beloved star of the '50s.

Kirk Douglas: A Hollywood Legend

Kirk Douglas's dynamic performances in films like "Spartacus," "Paths of Glory," and "Lust for Life" solidified his status as a Hollywood legend. His career spanned decades, leaving an enduring legacy.

It was a time of cinematic legends and iconic performances that continue to captivate audiences today. These actors and actresses defined an era of Hollywood glamour and artistry, leaving an indelible mark on the history of cinema. Their talent, charisma, and enduring appeal serve as a testament to the enduring power of storytelling through film.

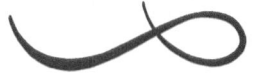

Innovation Unleashed - New Products

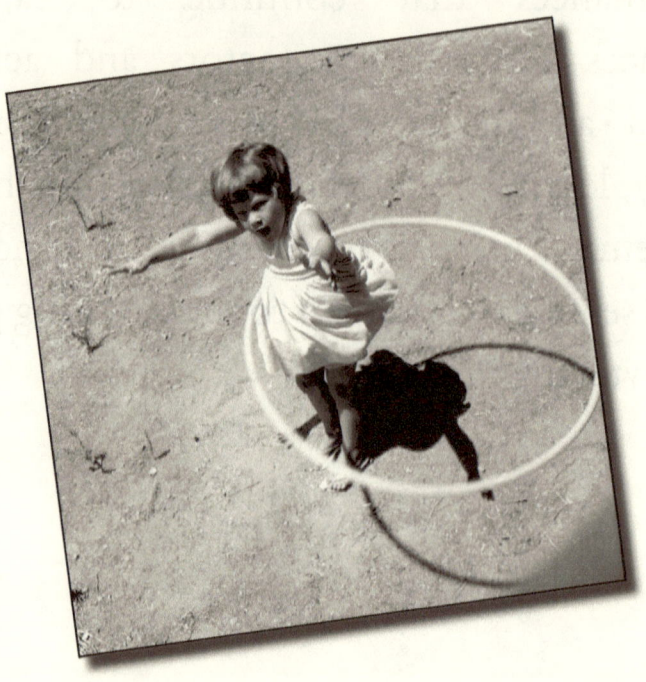

The 1950s was a decade of technological marvels and an insatiable appetite for all things new. America was buzzing with optimism and prosperity, and innovation was the name of the game. Its time to take a journey through some of the most exciting new products that shaped the American lifestyle and captured the spirit of the '50s.

The Television Set:
The Window to a New World

The 1950s was the decade when television truly came into its own. With the proliferation of television sets in homes across the country, families gathered around to watch programs like "I Love Lucy," "The Honeymooners," and "The Ed Sullivan Show." This magical box brought the world into living rooms and transformed entertainment forever.

The Frigidaire Refrigerator:
A Cool Revolution

The 1950s saw the widespread adoption of household appliances, and the Frigidaire refrigerator was at the forefront of this revolution. With improved refrigeration technology and sleek designs, these appliances made storing food more convenient and dependable.

The Microwave Oven:
A New Frontier in Cooking

In 1955, the first commercially successful microwave oven, the "Radarange," was introduced. This marvel of modern cooking technology allowed families to heat and cook food faster than ever before, changing meal preparation and convenience forever.

The Barbie Doll: A Toy for the Ages

In 1959, the world met Barbie, a fashion-forward doll that became an instant hit. Barbie brought the world of fashion and endless imaginative play into the lives of children, sparking creativity and dreams.

The Polaroid Camera: Instant Memories

The Polaroid camera, introduced in the late 1940s but reaching its peak in the 1950s, brought the magic of instant photography to the masses.

People could snap a picture and watch it develop before their eyes, capturing precious memories in seconds.

The Color TV: A Vibrant Upgrade

As the '50s progressed, black-and-white television sets made way for color TVs. With vibrant displays and a promise of brighter entertainment, color television enhanced the viewing experience and turned ordinary evenings into cinematic adventures.

The Chevy Corvette: An American Icon

In 1953, Chevrolet introduced the Corvette, a sleek sports car that epitomized the spirit of the open road. With its classic design and powerful engine, the Corvette became a symbol of American automotive prowess and passion.

The Jet Engine: A New Era of Air Travel

The development of jet engines in the 1950s revolutionized air travel. Commercial jetliners, like the Boeing 707, made long-distance travel faster and more accessible, shrinking the world and bringing people closer together.

The Iconic Diner: Where Food Meets Nostalgia

In the 1950s, diners became a staple of American culture. These quintessential eateries offered comfort food, milkshakes, and a nostalgic atmosphere that captured the essence of the era.

The Hula Hoop: Whirling into Fun

The Hula Hoop, invented in the late 1950s, became a sensation that swept the nation. This simple, plastic hoop brought joy and playful exercise to people of all ages.

The 1950s were a time of immense innovation and progress, and the products of that era reflect the spirit of an optimistic nation. Whether it was a new way to watch TV, a revolutionary kitchen appliance, or a sleek sports car, these products defined the decade and continue to influence our lives today. They were more than just items; they were symbols of a culture driven by the desire to explore new horizons, making the '50s a decade to remember.

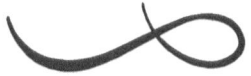

Timeless Tunes - Songs, Singers, and Bands

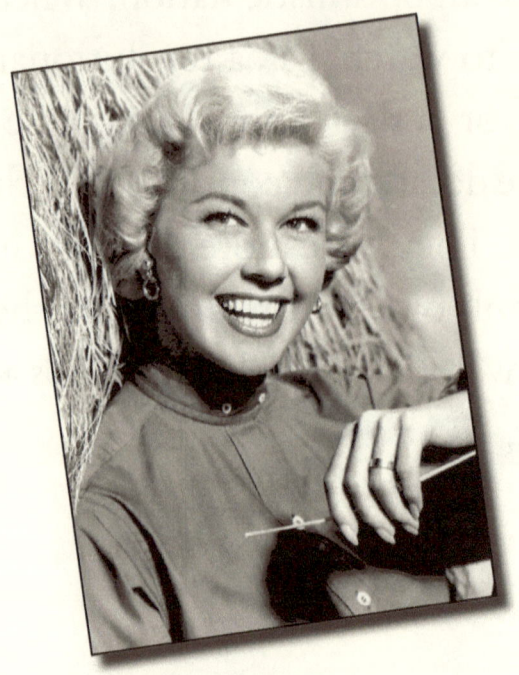

For America it was a time of musical magic, with legendary singers and iconic bands that left a lasting mark on the world of entertainment. It was an era of toe-tapping tunes and heartwarming ballads. In this article, let's take a friendly trip down the jukebox memory lane and revisit the famous songs, singers, and bands that rocked the '50s.

Rock 'n' Roll Revolution

The '50s saw the rise of rock 'n' roll, a genre that would forever change the music scene. Elvis Presley, often referred to as the "King of Rock 'n' Roll," became a household name with hits like "Heartbreak Hotel" and "Hound Dog." His hip-shaking performances and electrifying presence made him an instant sensation.

Buddy Holly and The Crickets

Buddy Holly and his band, The Crickets, brought us rock 'n' roll classics like "Peggy Sue" and "That'll Be the Day." Holly's distinctive glasses and infectious melodies made him an icon of the era.

Fats Domino: The Rhythm and Blues King

Fats Domino, known for hits like "Blueberry Hill" and "Ain't That a Shame," infused rhythm and blues with a New Orleans flair. His catchy piano tunes and warm vocals captured the hearts of listeners.

The Everly Brothers:
Close Harmony Perfection

The harmonious duo of Don and Phil Everly created timeless hits like "All I Have to Do Is Dream" and "Bye Bye Love." Their close harmonies and folk-inflected rock influenced generations of musicians.

The Birth of Doo-Wop

Doo-wop groups like The Platters, The Drifters, and The Five Satins brought soulful harmony to the airwaves. Hits like "Only You" and "Save the Last Dance for Me" provided the soundtrack to a generation in love.

Frank Sinatra: The Chairman of the Board

Frank Sinatra's smooth crooning style and impeccable phrasing made him an iconic figure. Songs like "My Way" and "Fly Me to the Moon" have become timeless classics, showcasing his enduring talent.

Nat King Cole: Unforgettable

Nat King Cole's velvety voice graced songs like "Unforgettable" and "Mona Lisa." He was a masterful pianist and a true gentleman of song.

Big Band Swing: The Duke and Count

The big band era found renewed life in the '50s with the Duke Ellington Orchestra and Count Basie's bands. Their swinging tunes like "Take the 'A' Train" and "April in Paris" kept the dance floors full.

Doris Day: America's Sweetheart of Song

Doris Day was not only a beloved actress but also a singer with hits like "Que Sera, Sera (Whatever Will Be, Will Be)" and "Secret Love." Her honeyed voice and heartfelt lyrics made her an American sweetheart.

The Golden Age of Doo-Wop

Doo-wop groups like The Coasters ("Yakety Yak"), The Chords ("Sh-Boom"), and The Crests ("Sixteen Candles") gave us harmonious gems that are still enjoyed today.

The 1950s were a time of musical legends and unforgettable melodies that continue to resonate through the decades. These singers and bands brought joy, nostalgia, and a sense of unity through their timeless tunes. They remind us that music has the power to transcend time, bringing people together and evoking emotions that are simply unforgettable.

See You Later, Aligator

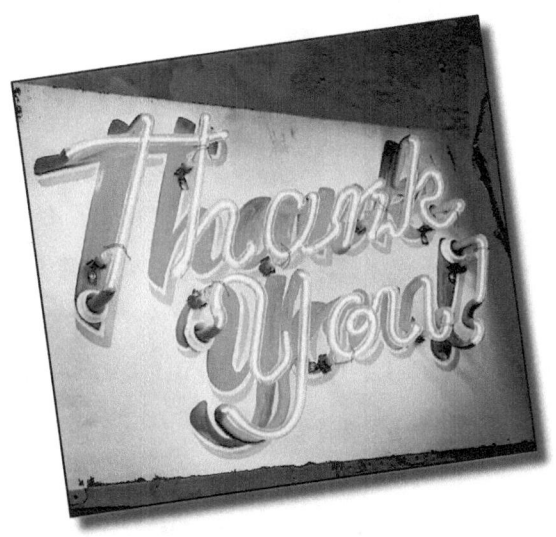

As we close the pages of our journey through 1950s America, let us linger a final moment in the glow of a neon sign and the sounds of a jukebox.

We've revisited the dawn of rock 'n' roll, history, fashion, sports, food, news, and more. We've witnessed a generation finding its voice.

Thank you, America.

Set in 18 pt EB Garamond
Copyright © 2023
Seniorality / Everbreeze Media Oy

seniorality.com
Quality Time for Seniors

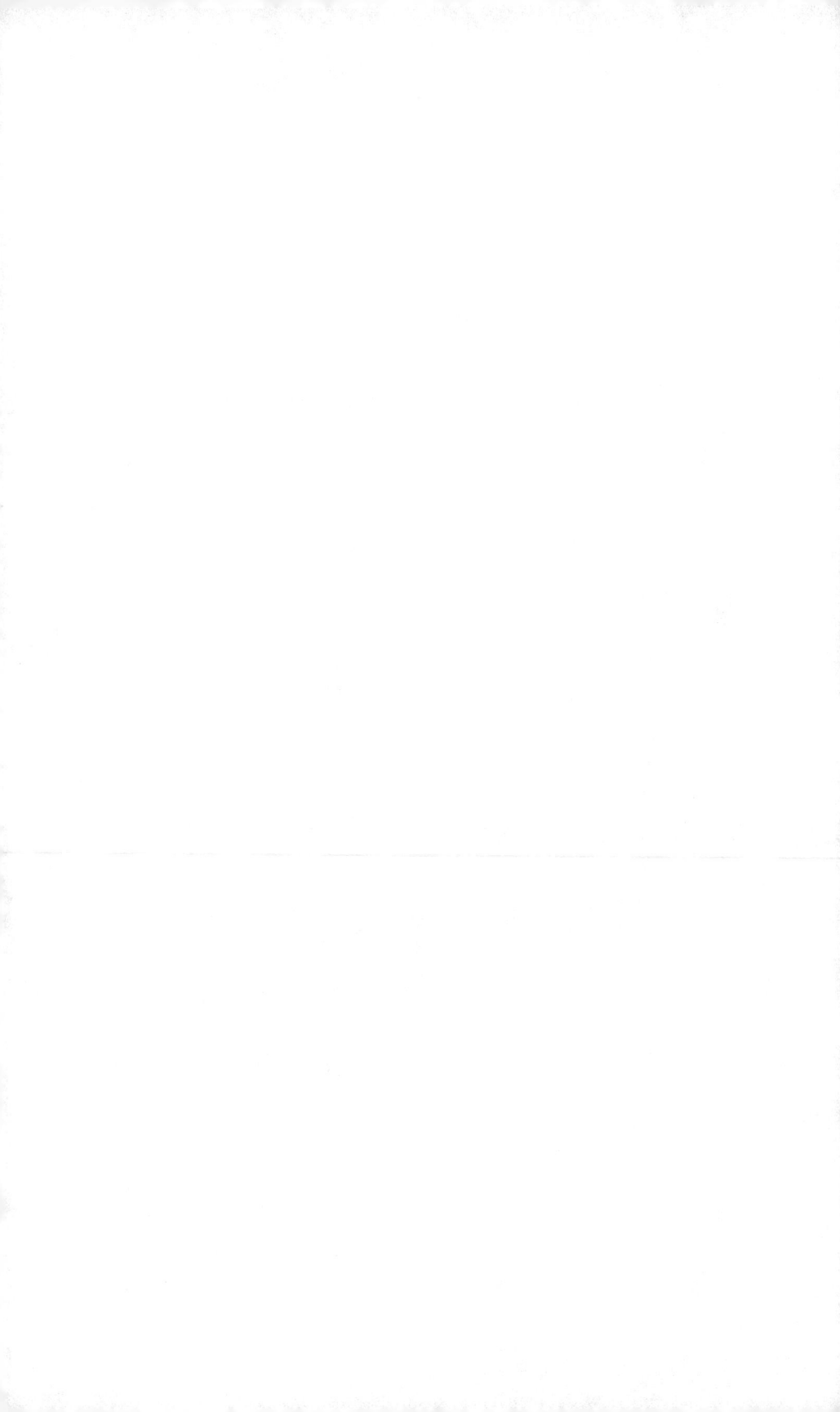

www.ingramcontent.com/pod-product-compliance
Lightning Source LLC
Chambersburg PA
CBHW020536290526
45786CB00002B/912